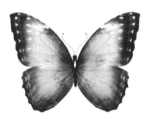

# My First
# Learn-to-Read
# Preschool
# Workbook

# FOR MY GIRLS.

-----------------------------

Series Designer: Stephanie Mautone
Interior and Cover Designer: Jami Splitter
Art Producer: Tom Hood
Editor: Julie Haverkate
Production Editor: Ashley Polikoff
Production Manager: Holly Haydash

All images used under license from iStockphoto.com and shutterstock.com

Paperback ISBN: 978-1-63878-143-1
R0

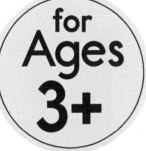

for Ages 3+

# MY FIRST
# Learn-to-Read
# Preschool
# WORKBOOK

## Practice Pre-Reading Skills *with* Phonics, Sight Words, and Simple Stories!

Sarah Chesworth

ROCKRIDGE
PRESS

# Note to Caregivers

Learning to read is one of the most magical milestones of childhood! *My First Learn-to-Read Preschool Workbook* will help your child begin this journey while making it fun, too. As a parent and teacher, I know the skills that will help kids prepare for school and set them up for success in the classroom . . . and beyond!

This book introduces some foundational reading concepts, including alphabet knowledge, phonemic awareness (the ability to hear sounds within a word), blending, critical thinking skills, fluency, and more!

Here are a few tips to ensure your child gets the most out of it:

- This book has been divided into four sections, which you should work through in order. At the beginning of each section, you will find a brief introduction and directions for guiding your child through the activities. These activities also include opportunities to build your child's vocabulary and expose them to foods, animals, and more!

- Go over each page with your child to ensure they know how to complete it.

- Take your time working through this book. Children learn at different speeds, and little learners may need multiple sessions to complete a page. Take breaks as needed and create a positive experience—kids learn best when they're having fun!

- Help your child make connections from the workbook to their world. For example, if they are working on a page about the letter A, ask them to look for objects in your home that begin with that letter.

Enjoy this special time as your child learns to read!

# Letter Sounds

● ○ ▲ ■ ▼ ○ ● ■ ● ○ ▲ ■ ▼ ○ ● ■ ● ○ ▲ ■ ▼ ○ ● ■ ● ○ ▲ ■

This section focuses on the letters of the alphabet and the sounds they represent. Your child will practice identifying each letter, writing it, and completing an activity with that letter sound. As you know, the English language is complex and there are always exceptions. Since this book is focused on the beginning reader, vowels will be introduced mostly using their short vowel sound. If your child is developmentally ready, you can discuss that sometimes vowels make a long sound. You can also explore how letters can be grouped together to make a different sound completely. Reading and writing go together, so your child will also practice writing letters. Each letter is introduced with numbers and arrows to help your child learn the proper way to write.

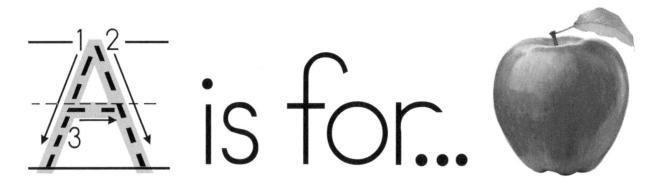

**A is for...**

Say and trace each letter.

Write the missing letter.

Circle the object that begins like the word **apple**.

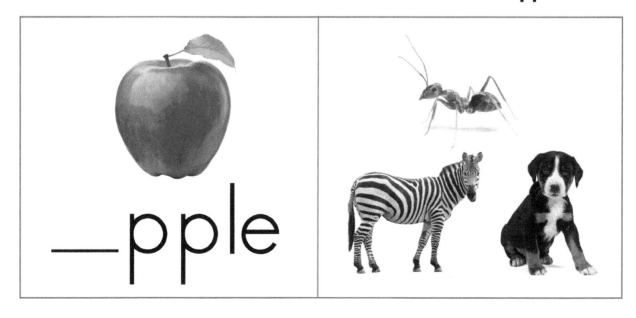

___pple

# B 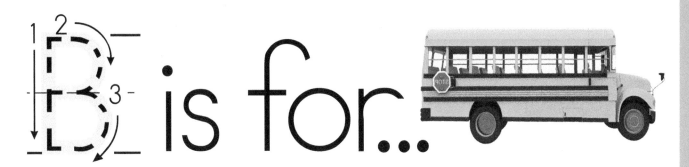 is for...

Say and trace each letter.

Write the missing letter.

Circle the objects that begin like the word **bus**.

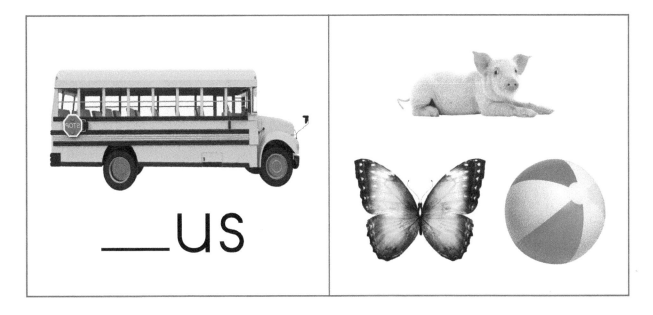

___us

C 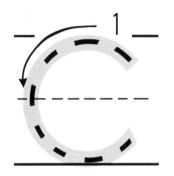 is for...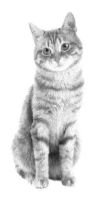

Say and trace each letter.

Write the missing letter.

Circle the objects that begin like the word **cat**.

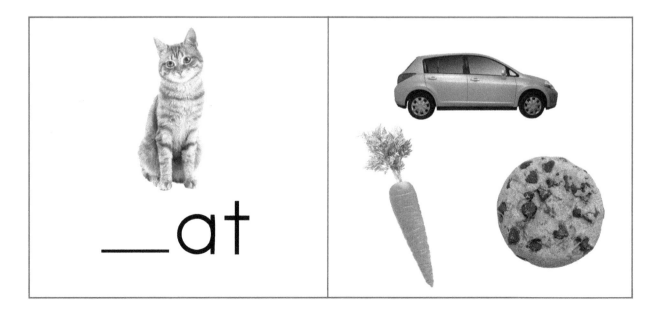

__at

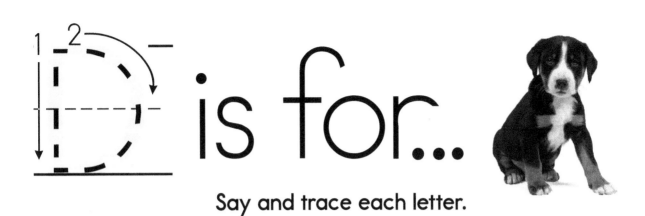

D is for...

Say and trace each letter.

Write the missing letter.

Circle the objects that begin like the word **dog**.

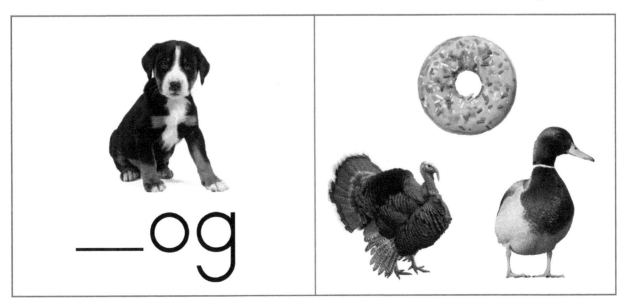

___og

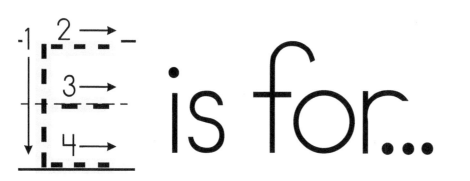 is for...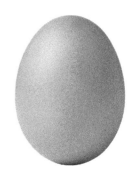

Say and trace each letter.

Write the missing letter.

Circle the object that begins
like the word **egg**.

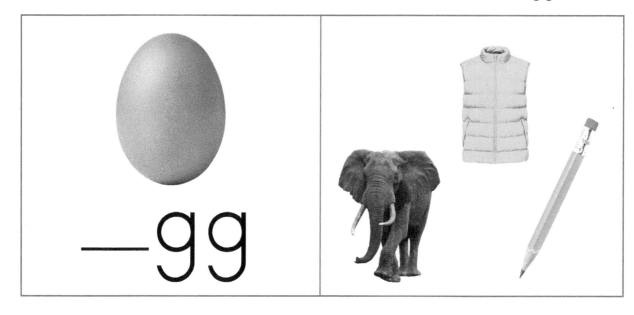

_gg

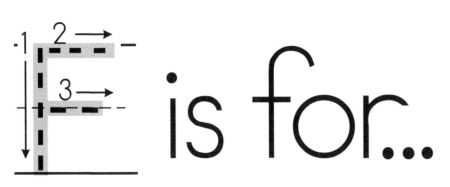 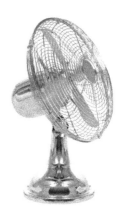

is for...

Say and trace each letter.

Write the missing letter.

Circle the objects that begin like the word **fan**.

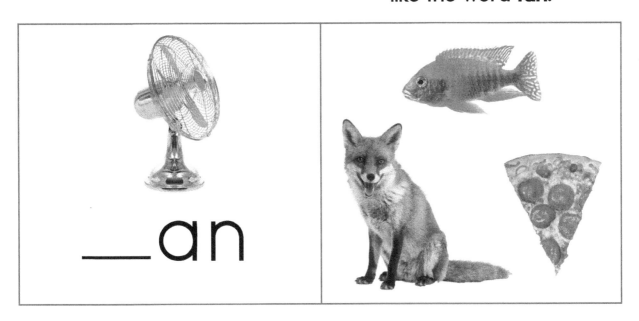

_an

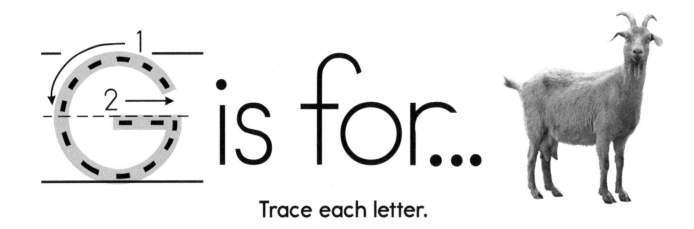 is for...

Trace each letter.

Write the missing letter.

Circle the object that begins like the word **goat**.

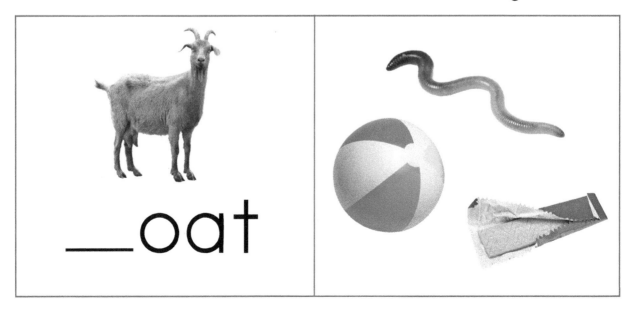

_oat

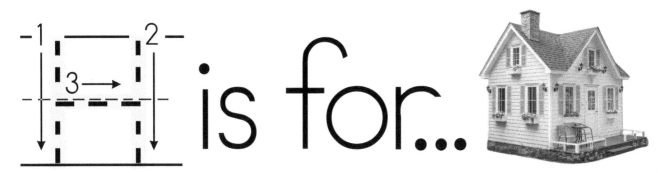 is for...

Say and trace each letter.

Write the missing letter.

Circle the objects that begin like the word **house**.

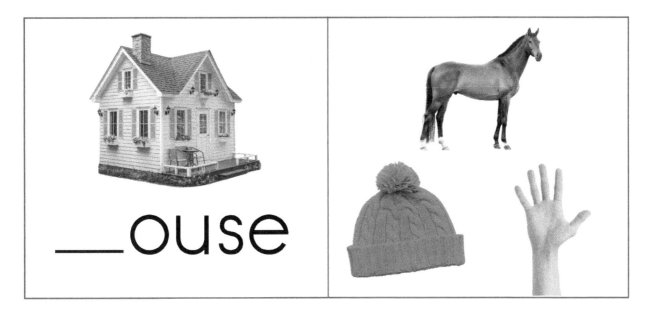

__ouse

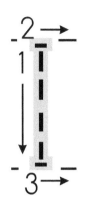

# I is for...

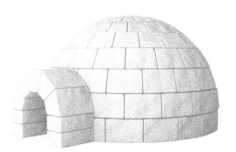

Say and trace each letter.

Write the missing letter.

Circle the object that begins like the word **igloo**.

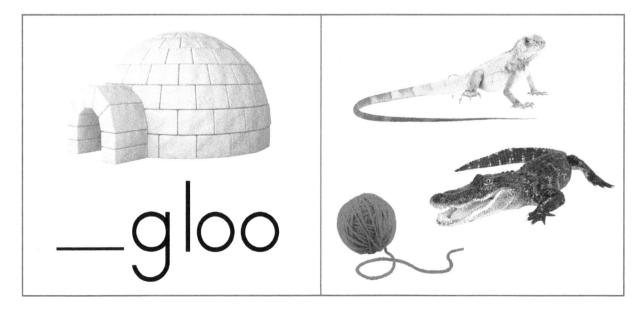

__gloo

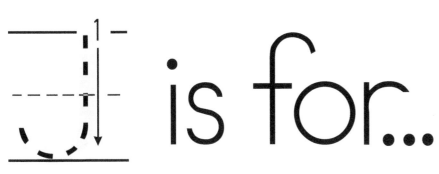 is for...

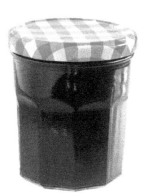

Say and trace each letter.

Write the missing letter.

Circle the objects that begin like the word **jam**.

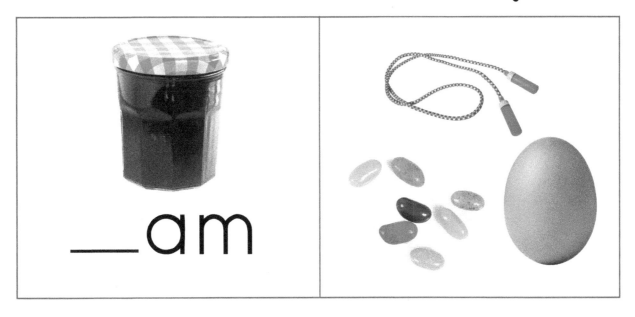

___am

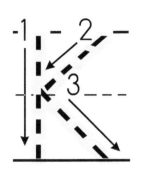 **K** is for...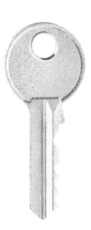

Say and trace each letter.

Write the missing letter.

Circle the object that begins like the word **key**.

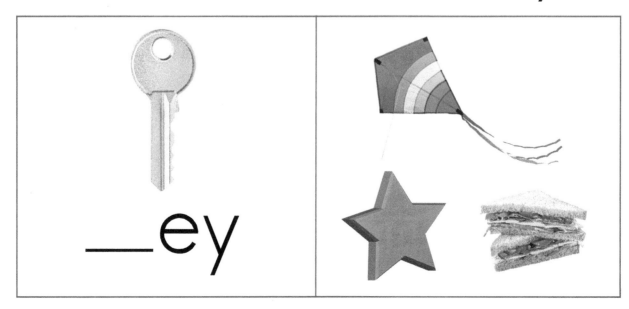

__ey

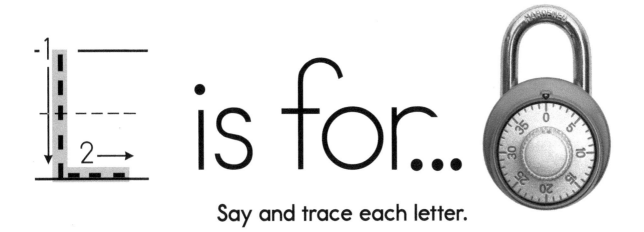

# L is for...

Say and trace each letter.

Write the missing letter.

Circle the objects that begin like the word **lock**.

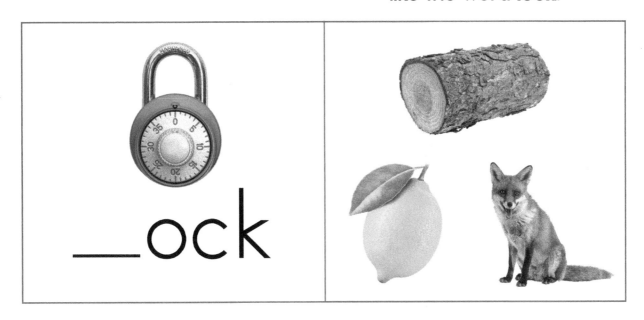

__ock

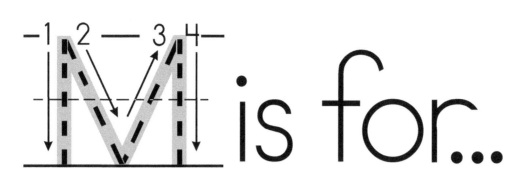 **is for...**

Say and trace each letter.

Write the missing letter.

Circle the object that begins like the word **mop**.

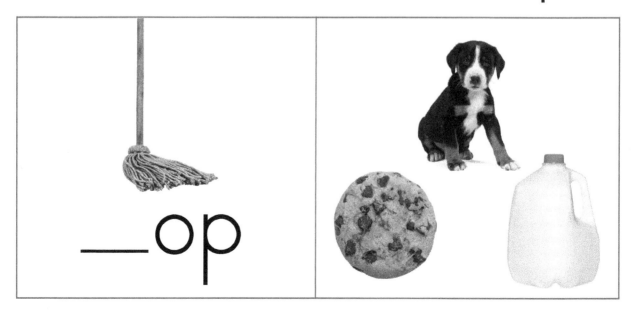

__op

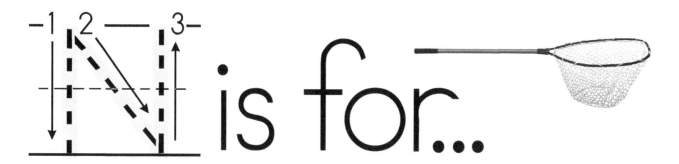

# N is for...

Say and trace each letter.

Write the missing letter.

Circle the objects that begin like the word **net**.

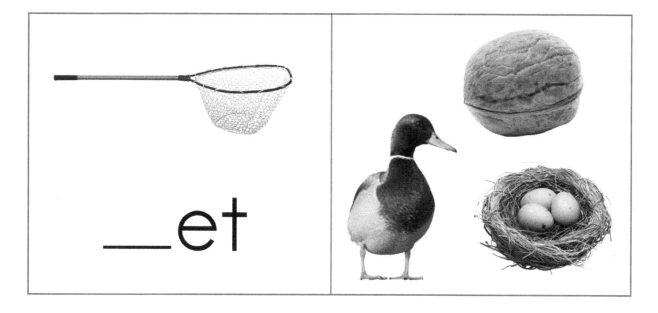

__et

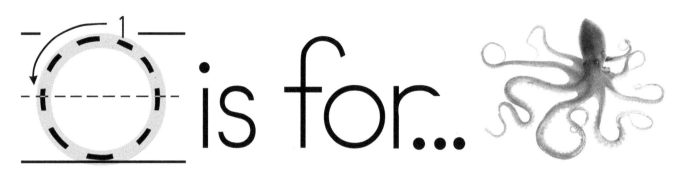

# O is for...

Say and trace each letter.

Write the missing letter.

Circle the object that begins like the word **octopus**.

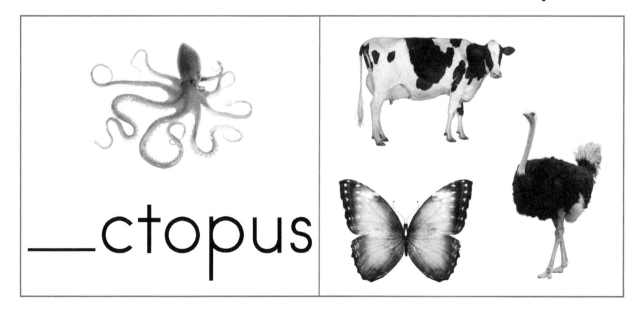

__ctopus

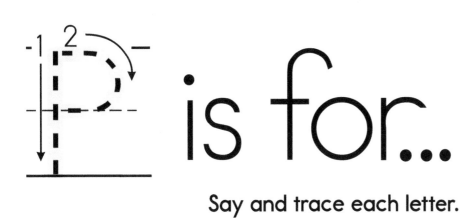

# P is for...

Say and trace each letter.

Write the missing letter.

Circle the objects that begin like the word **pencil**.

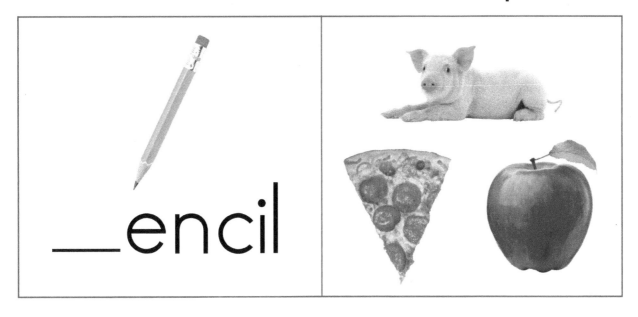

__encil

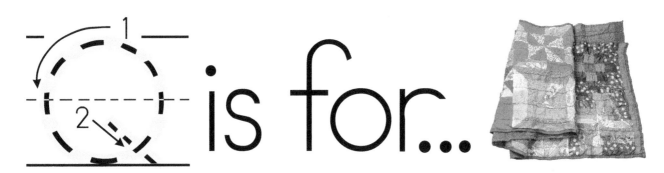 is for...

Say and trace each letter.

Write the missing letter.

Circle the object that begins like the word **quilt**.

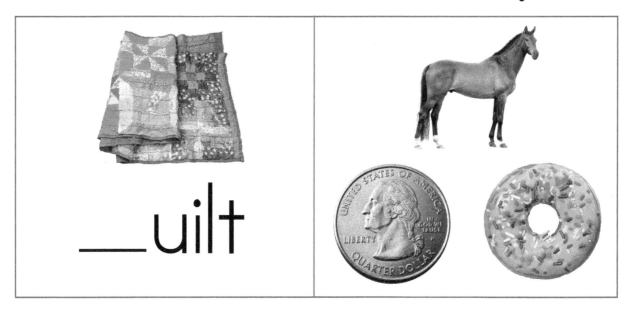

__uilt

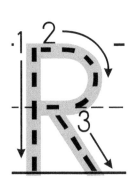 **R** is for...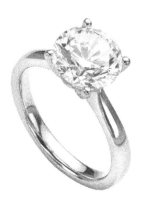

Say and trace each letter.

Write the missing letter.

Circle the objects that begin like the word **ring**.

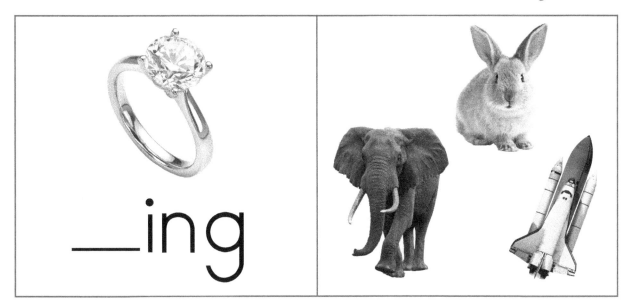

___ing

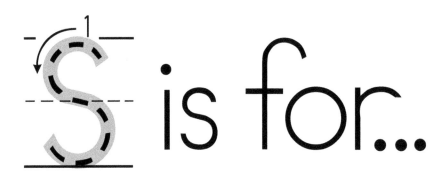 is for...

Say and trace each letter.

Write the missing letter.

Circle the objects that begin like the word **sand.**

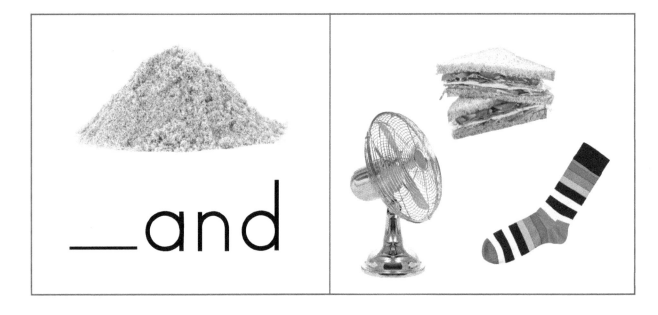

__and

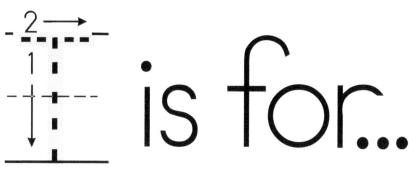 is for...

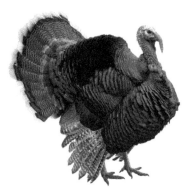

Say and trace each letter.

Write the missing letter.

Circle the objects that begin like the word **turkey**.

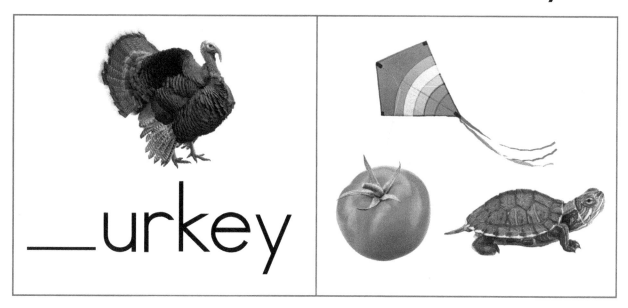

___urkey

U is for...

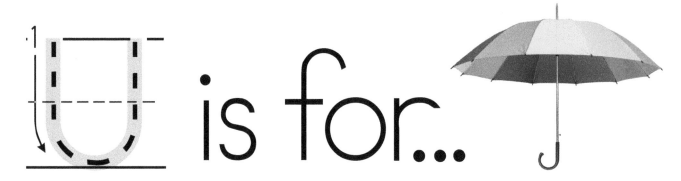

Say and trace each letter.

Write the missing letter.

Circle the object that begins like the word **umbrella**.

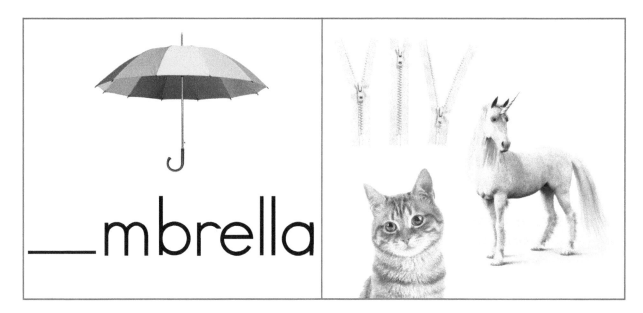

__mbrella

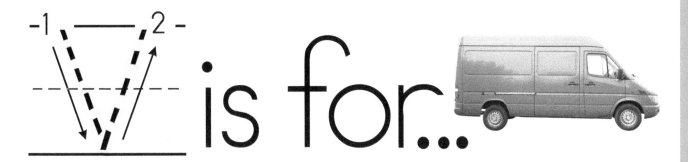

V is for...

## Say and trace each letter.

Write the missing letter.

Circle the object that begins like the word **van**.

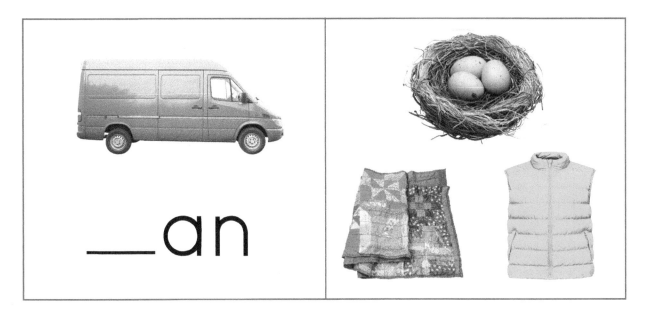

__an

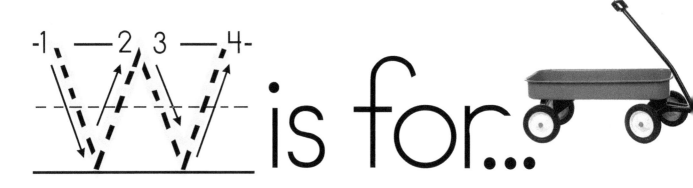

W is for...

Say and trace each letter.

Write the missing letter.

Circle the objects that begin like the word **wagon**.

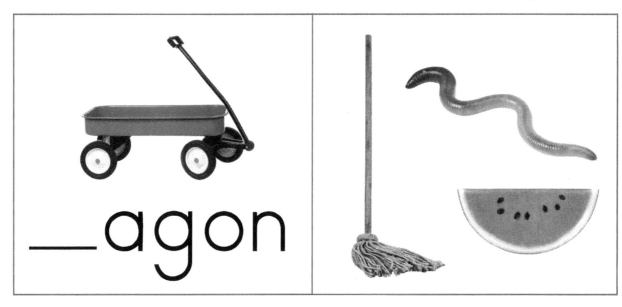

__agon

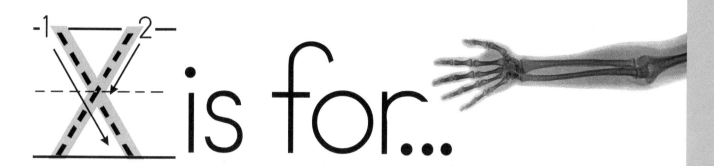

# X is for...

Say and trace each letter.

Write the missing letter.

Circle the objects that end with the letter **X**.

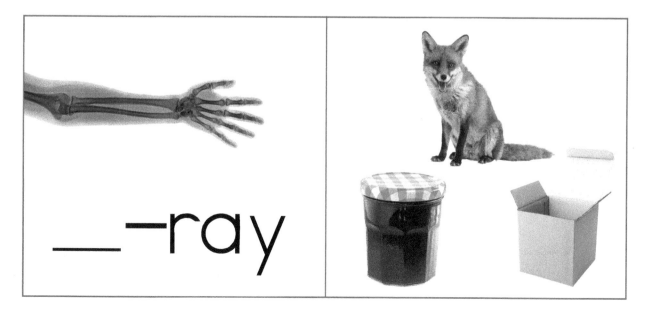

___−ray

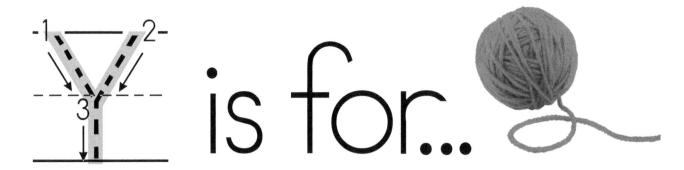

# Y is for...

Say and trace each letter.

Write the missing letter.

Circle the object that begins like the word **yarn**.

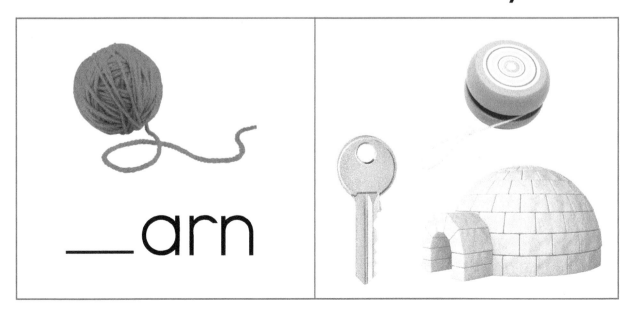

__arn

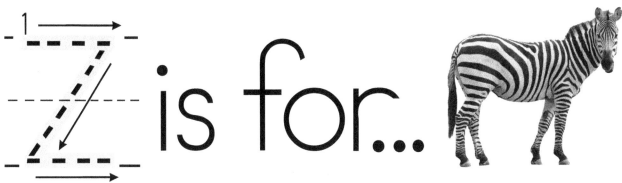

# Z is for...

Say and trace each letter.

Write the missing letter.

Circle the object that begins like the word **zebra**.

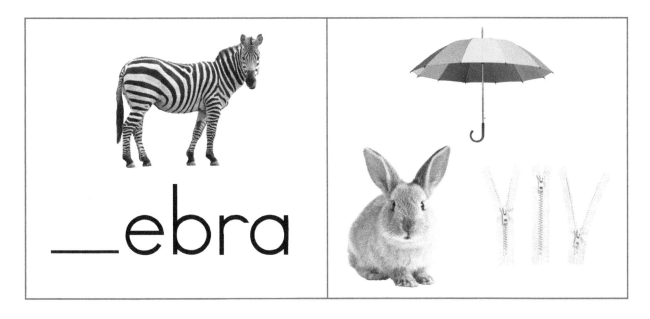

__ebra

# Show What You Know

Draw a line from each picture to its beginning letter.

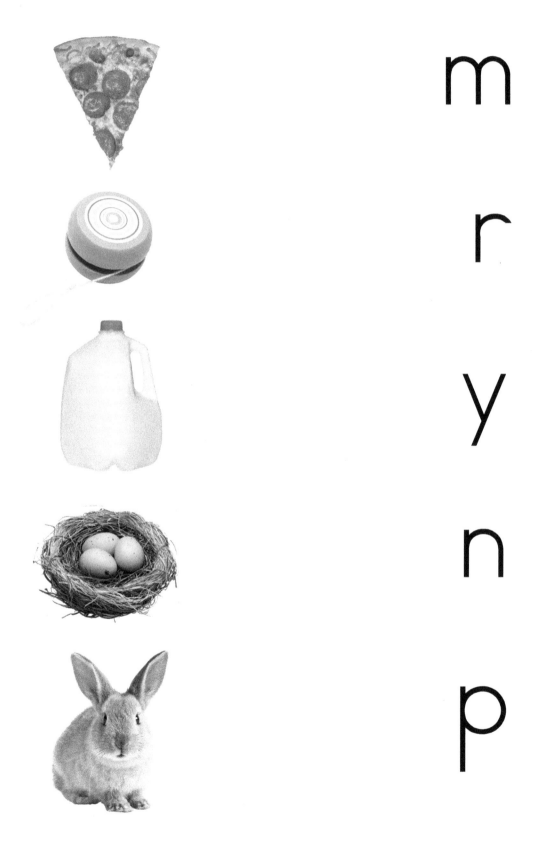

m

r

y

n

p

# Make a Word

Write each missing letter to complete the words.

| j v d f |

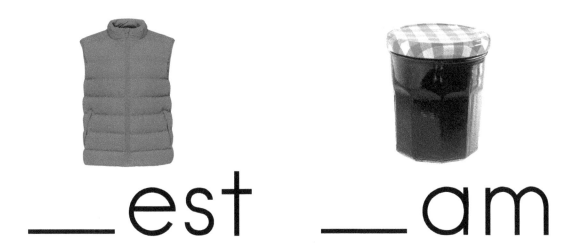

___est        ___am

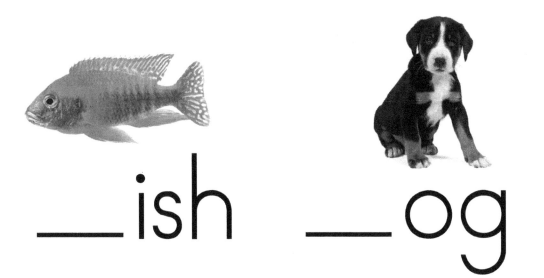

___ish        ___og

# Same Sounds

Circle the words that begin or end with **g**.

dog

six

gum

get

log

net

can

web

leg

rat

# Circle It!

Circle the words that begin the same
as the picture in each row.

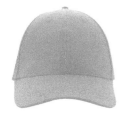 cub rag cat pen

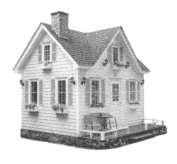 hit hug van fun

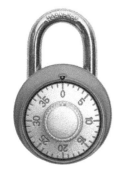 log ran leg pig

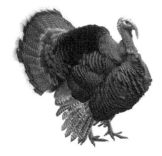 tap dog ten tan

# Word Hunt

Find and circle each word in the puzzle.

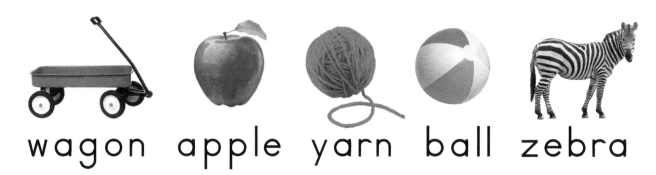

wagon    apple    yarn    ball    zebra

| a | p | p | l | e | j |
|---|---|---|---|---|---|
| p | b | a | s | t | h |
| d | w | a | g | o | n |
| y | a | r | n | k | q |
| e | z | e | b | r | a |
| f | g | b | a | l | l |

# Blending Sounds

●○▲■▼○■●○▲■▼○■●○▲■▼○■●○▲■

In this section, your little one will start reading simple words. As they complete the activities, encourage them to think of other words that follow the same patterns.

First, your child will learn consonant-vowel-consonant (CVC) words in common word families. Word families help beginning readers see patterns within words. You can also point out that when words sound the same at the end, they rhyme!

Next, your child will move on to blends and digraphs. A blend is when two letters make a sound together, but each letter sound can still be heard. For example, **bl** as in *block*. A digraph is when two letters represent one sound together, like **sh** in *fish*. There are many more blends and digraphs than this book can cover, but a few of the most common ones have been chosen to introduce the concept.

# -ap Word Family as in...

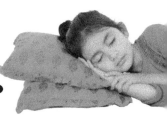

Trace all the letters. Then say each sound and word.

Write the missing letters.

Circle the objects that end like the word **nap**.

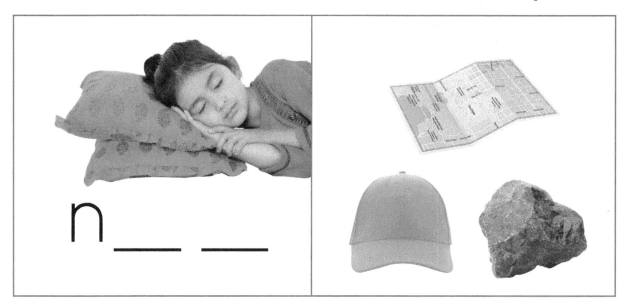

n___ ___

# -at Word Family as in...

Trace all the letters. Then say each sound and word.

Write the missing letters.

Circle the objects that end like the word **bat**.

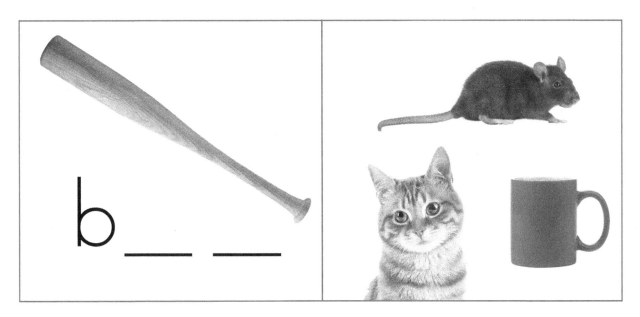

b __ __

# -ed Word Family as in...

Trace all the letters. Then say each sound and word.

Write the missing letters.    Circle the object that ends like the word **bed**.

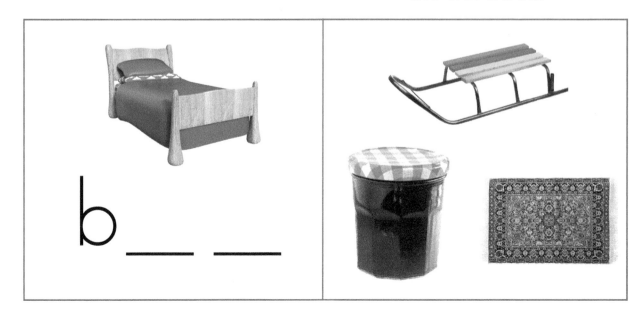

# -et Word Family as in...

Trace all the letters. Then say each sound and word.

Write the missing letters.

Circle the objects that end like the word **jet**.

j___ ___

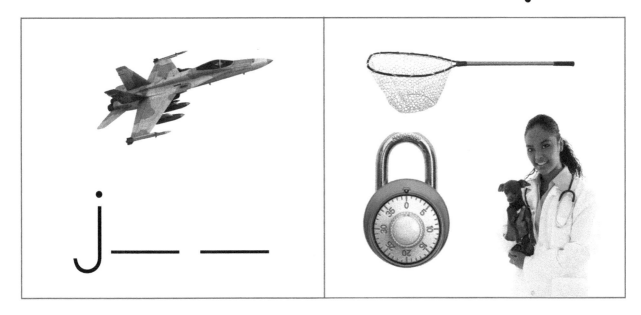

# -ig Word Family as in...

Trace all the letters. Then say each sound and word.

Write the missing letters.

Circle the object that ends like the word **pig**.

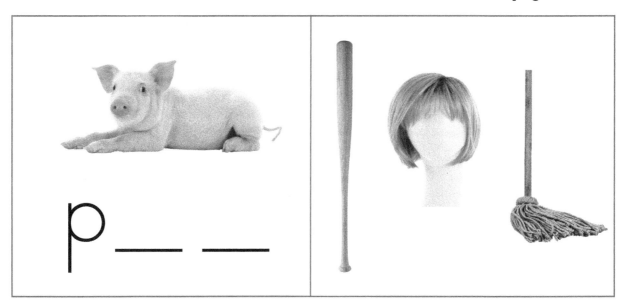

p＿ ＿

# -ock Word Family as in...

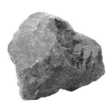

Trace all the letters. Then say each sound and word.

Write the missing letters.

Circle the objects that end like the word **rock**.

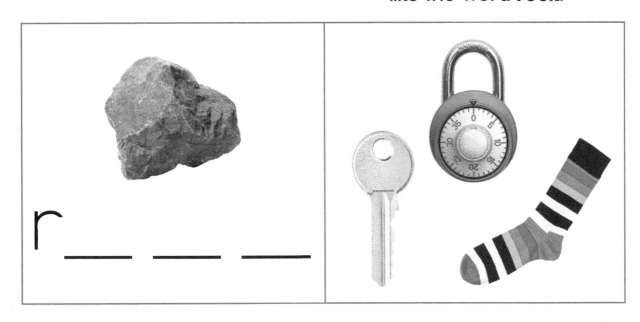

r_ _ _ _

# -ug Word Family as in...

Trace all the letters. Then say each sound and word.

Write the missing letters.

Circle the objects that end like the word **bug**.

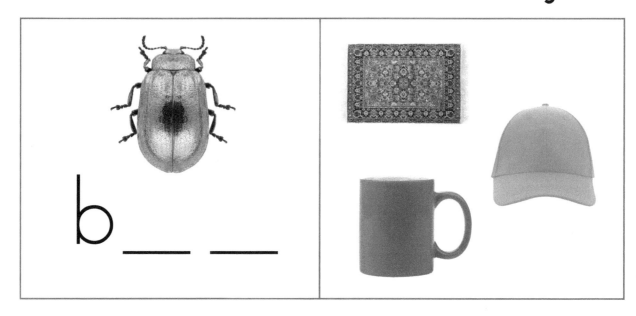

b __ __

# -un Word Family as in...

Trace all the letters. Then say each sound and word.

Write the missing letters.

Circle the object that ends like the word **bun**.

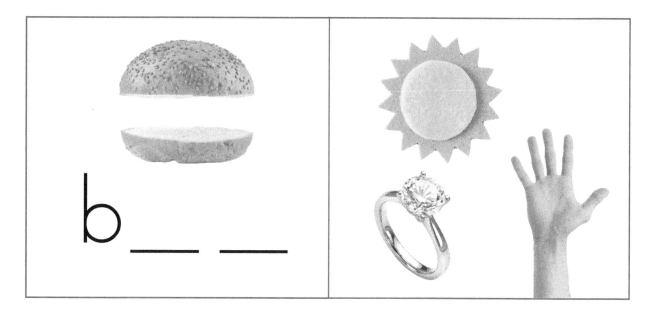

# bl- Blend as in...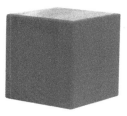

Trace all the letters. Then say each sound and word.

Write the missing letters.

Circle the objects that begin like the word **block**.

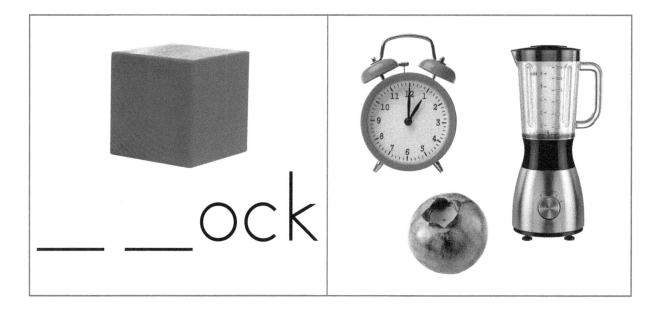

___ ___ock

# fr- Blend as in...

Trace all the letters. Then say each sound and word.

Write the missing letters.

Circle the objects that begin like the word **frog**.

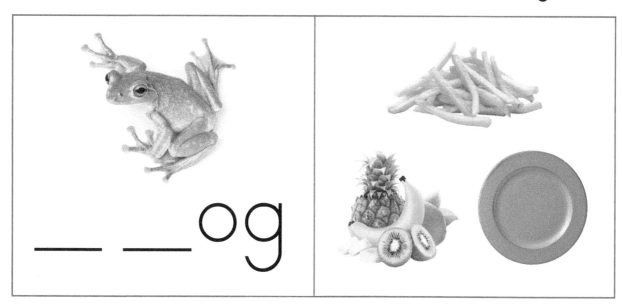

___ ___og

# sn- Blend as in...

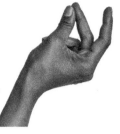

Trace all the letters. Then say each sound and word.

Write the missing letters.

Circle the objects that begin like the word **snap.**

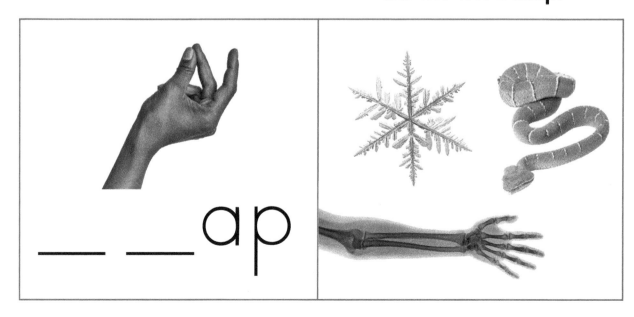

___ ___ ap

# ch- Digraph as in...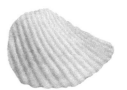

Trace all the letters. Then say each sound and word.

Write the missing letters.

Circle the objects that begin like the word **chip.**

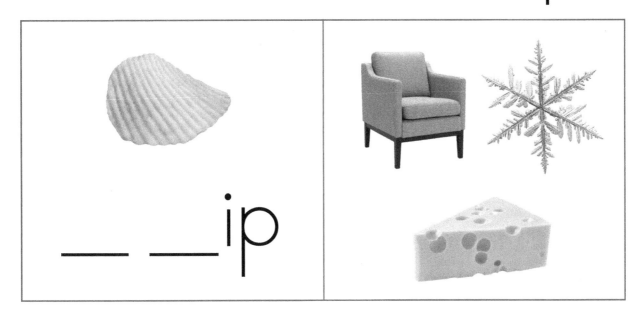

__ __ip

# -sh Digraph as in...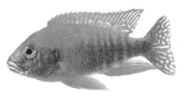

Trace all the letters. Then say each sound and word.

Write the missing letters.

Circle the objects that end like the word **fish**.

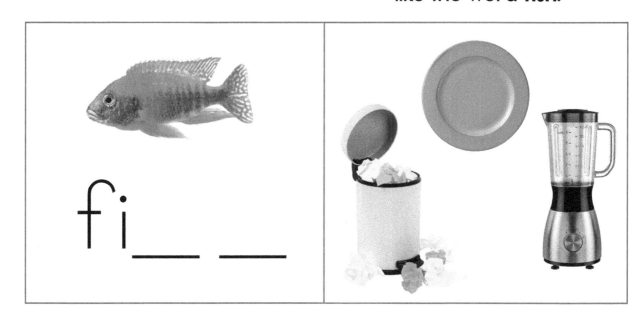

fi_ _

# -th Digraph as in...

Trace all the letters. Then say each sound and word.

Write the missing letters.

Circle the objects that end like the word **bath**.

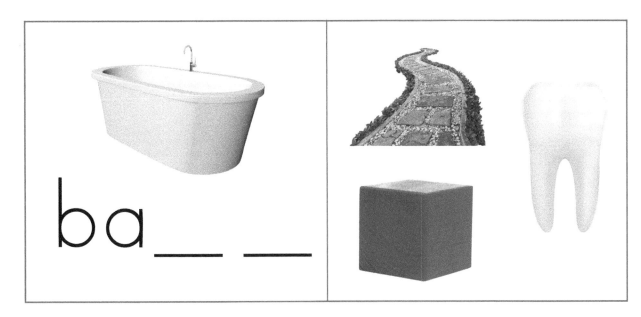

ba__ __

# Show What You Know

Draw a line from each picture to the matching word.

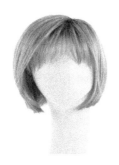

r u g

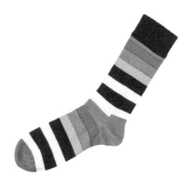

s o c k

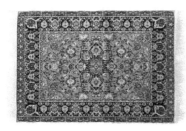

m a p

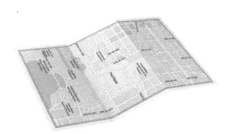

w i g

# Make a Word

Write the missing letters to complete each word.

| fr sh th bl |

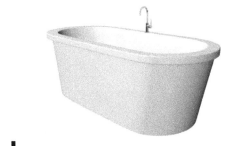

ba_ _ _

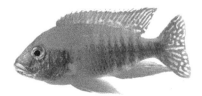

fi_ _ _

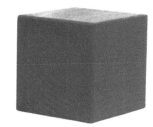

_ _ _ock

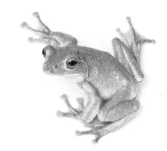

_ _ _og

# Same Sounds

Circle the words that begin or end with **sh**.

bath

ship

chip

wish

thin

dish

shock

chop

fish

path

# Circle It!

Circle the words that rhyme with
the picture in each row.

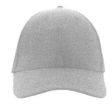 rap tap cat wet

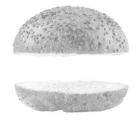 wed fun run bat

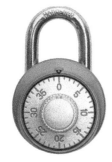 sock tug flock dig

set slug met nap

# Word Hunt

Find and circle each word in the puzzle.

snap      fish      jet      block      bat

| b | a | t | g | r | e |
|---|---|---|---|---|---|
| o | m | x | j | e | t |
| p | b | l | o | c | k |
| c | n | s | n | w | y |
| f | s | n | a | p | z |
| d | v | f | i | s | h |

# Sight Words

Now that your child has practiced with letters, blends, and word families, they can progress to reading sight words. Sight words often don't follow normal phonemic patterns. That means children learn to read them by sight rather than sounding out the letters individually. These are the most common words in texts, and they usually aren't linked to a concrete image. Knowing these words will help build your child's reading fluency and confidence!

There are many more sight words than this book can cover, so a few of the most common ones have been chosen. Repetition is key to learning these words. Have your child read each page multiple times and encourage them to look for these words in other books, too!

# Sight Word: Go

I can go home.

Trace and say each word.

Write the missing letters to make the word **go**.

# Circle each balloon that has the word **go**.

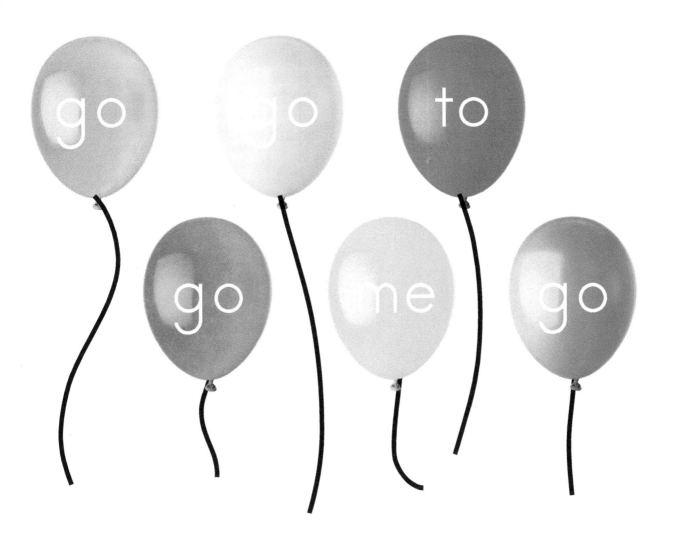

## Write the missing word to complete the sentence.

I can ⬜⬜ home.

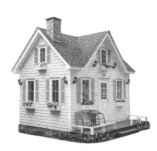

# Sight Word: To

I like **to** read.

Trace and say each word.

Write the missing letters to make the word **to**.

Circle each book that has the word **to**.

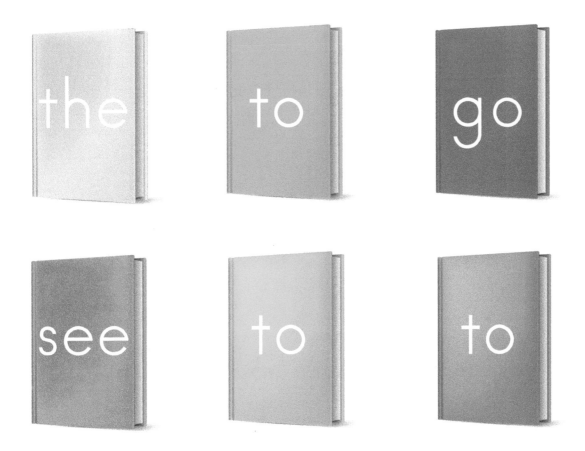

Write the missing word to complete the sentence.

I like ☐☐ read.

# Sight Word: Is

This | is | my pet dog.

Trace and say each word.

Write the missing letters to make the word **is**.

## Circle each star that has the word **is**.

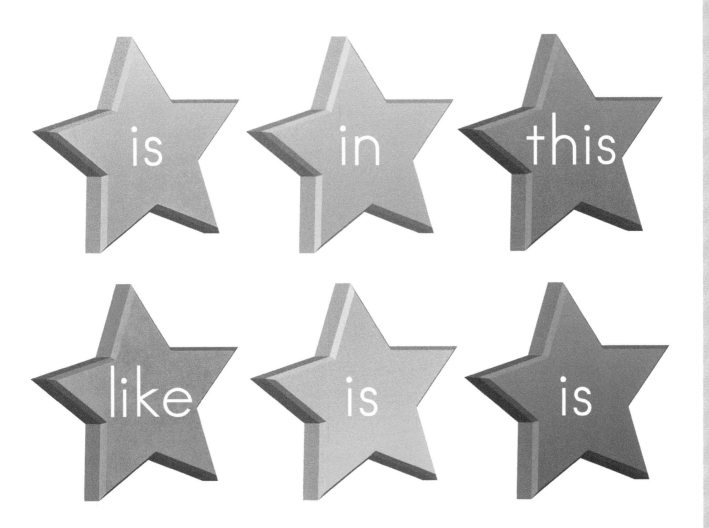

is    in    this

like    is    is

## Write the missing word to complete the sentence.

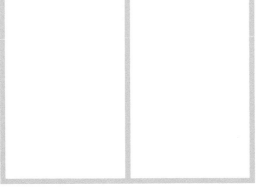

This ☐☐ my pet dog.

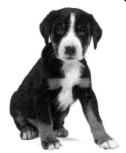

# Sight Word: My

This is  m y  bus.

Trace and say each word.

Write the missing letters to make the word **my**.

Circle each tire that has the word **my**.

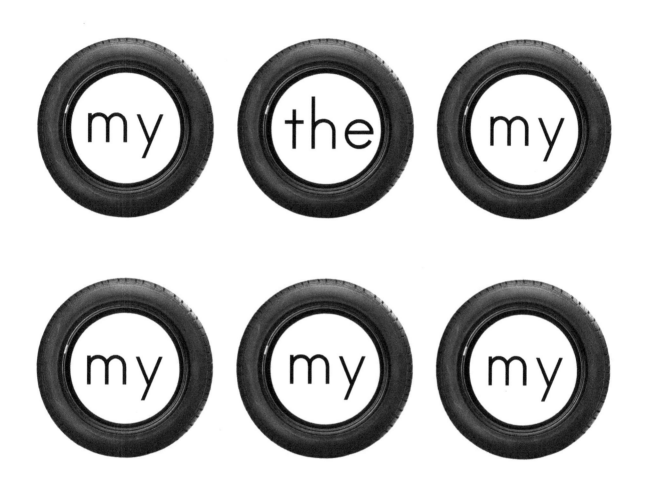

Write the missing word to complete the sentence.

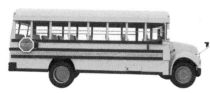

This is ☐☐ bus.

# Sight Word: See

I can see a bug.

Trace and say each word.

Write the missing letters to make the word **see**.

Circle each flower that has the word **see**.

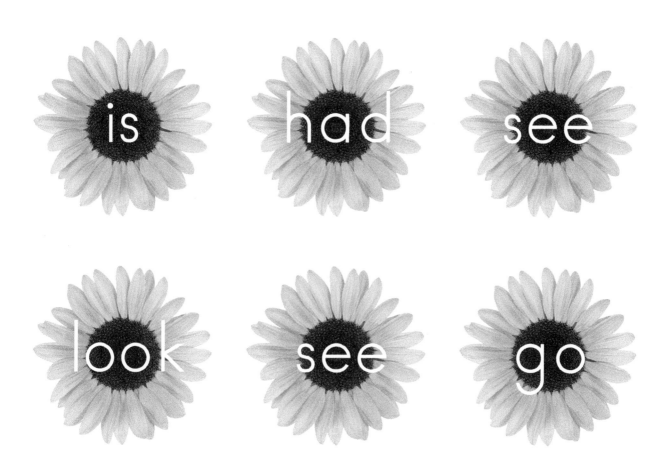

is    had    see

look    see    go

Write the missing word to complete the sentence.

I can ⬚⬚⬚ a bug.

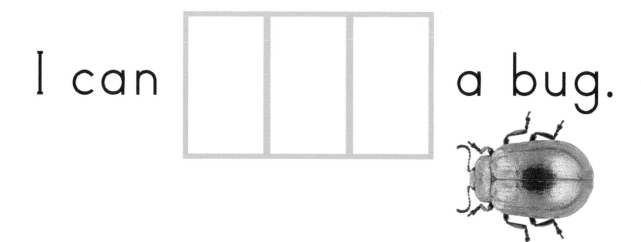

# Sight Word: The

We can go to the beach.

Trace and say each word.

Write the missing letters to make the word **the.**

# Circle each bucket that has the word **the**.

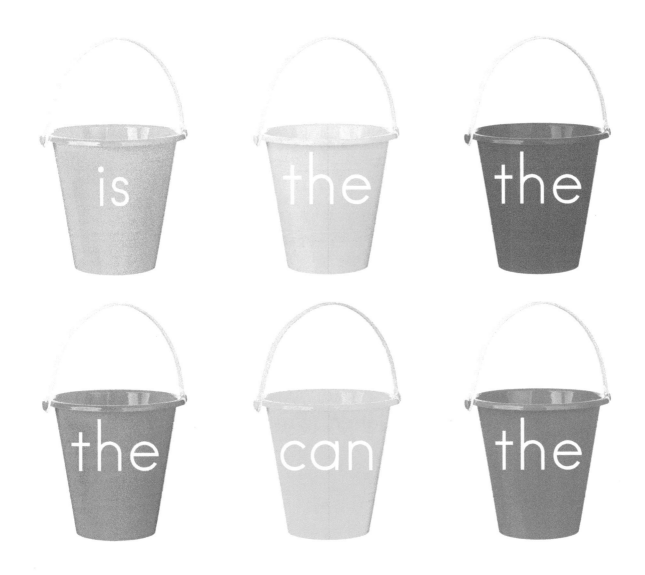

is    the    the

the    can    the

Write the missing word to complete the sentence.

We can go to ▭▭▭ beach.

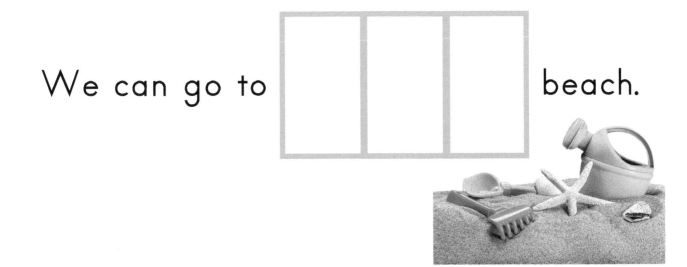

# Sight Word: You

I love you.

Trace and say each word.

Write the missing letters to make the word **you**.

Circle each heart that has the word **you**.

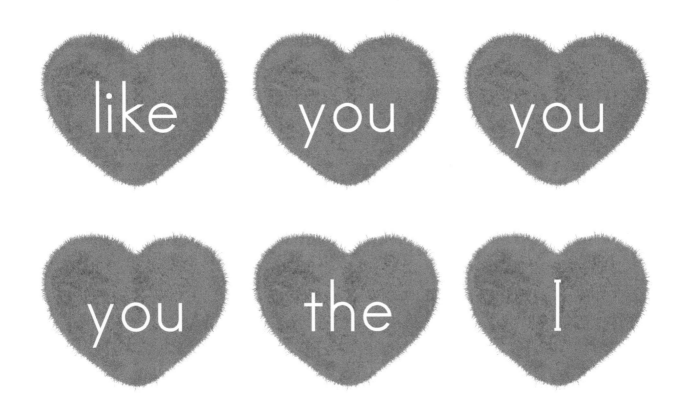

like    you    you

you    the    I

Write the missing word to complete the sentence.

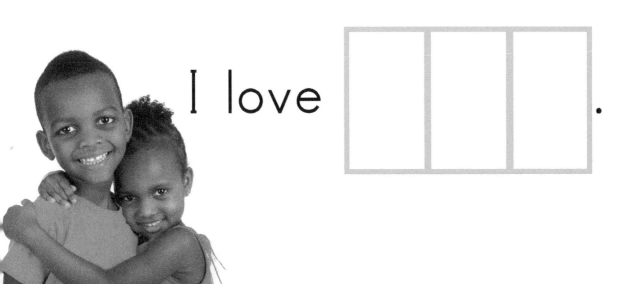

I love ⬚⬚⬚.

# Sight Word: Like

I  like  cookies.

Trace and say each word.

Write the missing letters to make the word **like**.

Circle each cookie that has the word **like**.

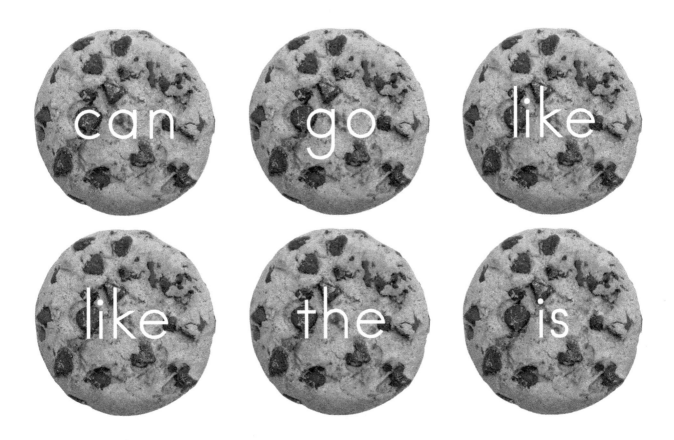

Write the missing word to complete the sentence.

I | | | | cookies.

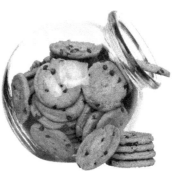

# Sight Word: And

I like milk  and  cookies.

Trace and say each word.

Write the missing letters to make the word **and**.

Circle each bottle of milk that has the word **and**.

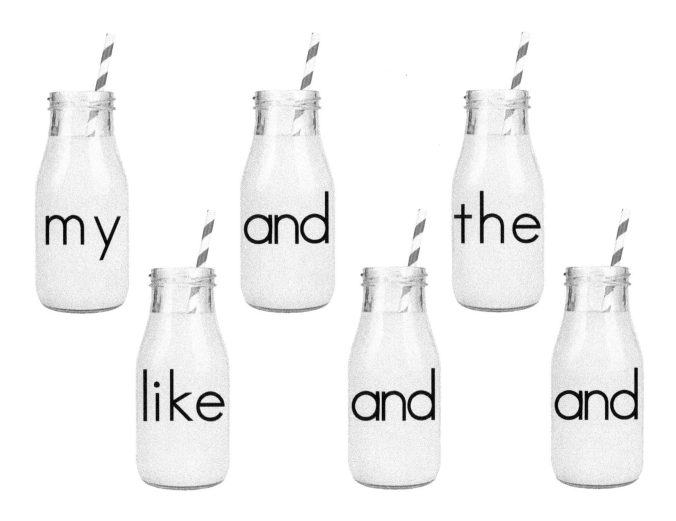

Write the missing word to complete the sentence.

I like milk ☐☐☐ cookies.

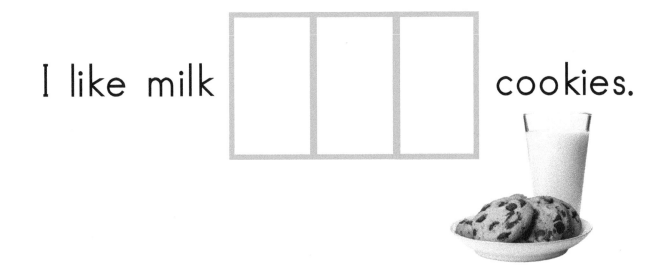

# Word Hunt

Find and circle each word in the puzzle.

| | | | | | |
|---|---|---|---|---|---|
| and | to | my | see | you | |

| | | | | | |
|---|---|---|---|---|---|
| t | h | s | e | e | l |
| d | s | w | y | o | u |
| a | n | d | h | b | k |
| l | g | n | t | o | p |
| t | w | z | r | m | y |
| r | o | c | e | f | a |

| | | | | | |
|---|---|---|---|---|---|
| go | is | the | like | this | |

| | | | | | |
|---|---|---|---|---|---|
| w | o | p | g | i | s |
| f | t | h | i | s | k |
| s | e | g | o | o | l |
| l | p | a | g | s | c |
| t | h | e | h | f | d |
| q | l | i | k | e | z |

# Simple Stories

● ▲ ■ ▼ ● ■ ● ■ ● ▲ ■ ▼ ● ■ ● ■ ● ▲ ■ ▼ ● ■ ● ■ ● ▲ ■

The stories in this section focus on word families and sight words previously introduced in this book. Your child will practice reading these simple stories and completing an activity to go with each one. This will give them experience decoding words, while also boosting their confidence!

As you work through this final section:

- Remember reading should be a fun and positive experience! If your child is frustrated, stop and take a break.

- Encourage your child to point to each word as they read. This helps your child understand that each written word is also a spoken word.

- Point out the punctuation to your child and model how to pause at the end of the sentence when you see a period.

- Have your child read each story multiple times to increase reading fluency.

- Ask your child simple comprehension questions. A comprehension activity is included with each story.

# Pat the Cat:
# -at Word Family

Pat is a fat cat. He sat on a hat. The hat is flat. That cat!

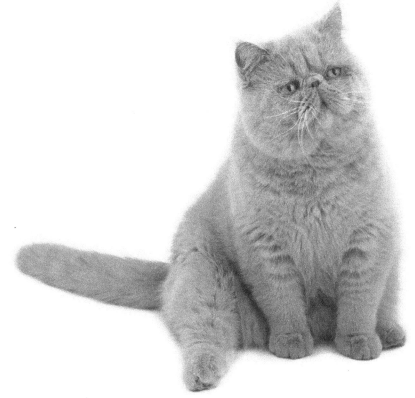

Draw a picture of what Pat sat on.

# Same Sounds

Circle each word in the **-at** family and read it aloud.

hat

sat

cat

can flat

is

jet

fat

that

red

on

pat

# A Fish Wish:
# -sh Digraph

The fish made a wish. The wish is to see a ship.
But the ship is in the shed. The fish is sad.

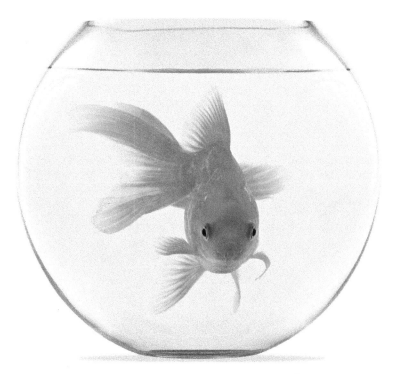

Draw a picture of the fish's wish.

# Same Sounds

Circle the words that begin or end with **sh**.

wish

sad

ship

the chop

bath

shed

fish

shop

math

chip

is

# My Pets: Sight Words

I like my rat. I like my frog. I like my cat.
I like my pig. I love my dog!

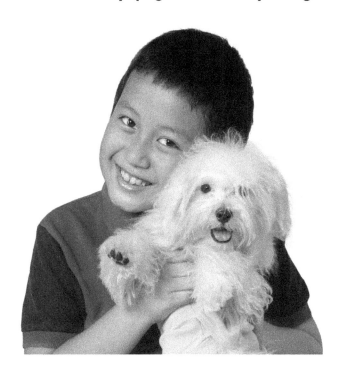

Draw a picture of one pet.

# Same Sounds

How many times can you find each sight word?
Count the words and write the number.

☐ ☐ ☐

I    like    my

I

like    my

I

sat

like

like    my

my

# Go:
# Sight Words

You can see the van go. You can see the bus go.
You can see the jet go fast!

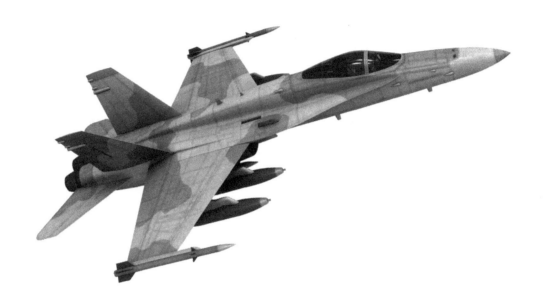

Draw a picture of one object that can go.

# Same Sounds

How many times can you find each sight word?
Count the words and write the number.

| | | |
|---|---|---|
| ☐ | ☐ | ☐ |
| you | can | see |
| ☐ | ☐ | ☐ |
| the | go | my |

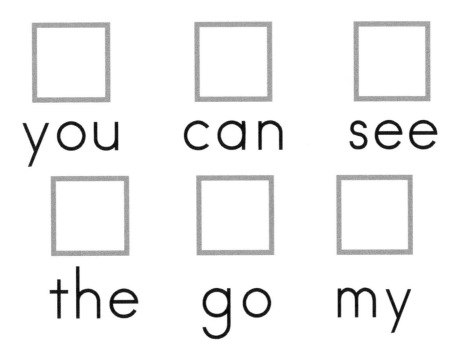

go my you
go see go my
the can the
go the
my can

# On Your Way!

Use the code to discover a secret message!

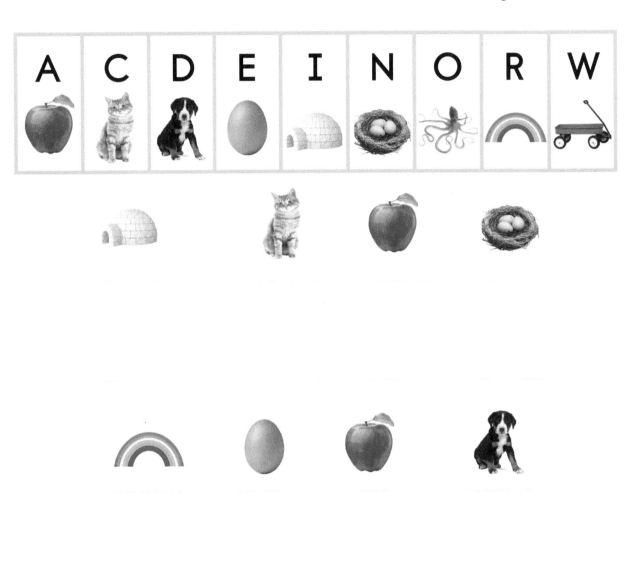

ICAN

WEDO

NOW!

# This certificate is presented to

for learning to read!

_____
Date

# About the Author

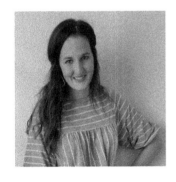

**Sarah Chesworth** is a former kindergarten and first grade teacher. Now she spends her days teaching her own two little girls. She also helps busy parents and teachers make learning fun through her website and online teaching resources at sarahchesworth.com. She holds a bachelor's degree in early childhood education from Texas Tech University.

CPSIA information can be obtained
at www.ICGtesting.com
Printed in the USA
JSHW040151131022
31601JS00002B/2